LIVE IT UP!

SHARE A GREAT LIFE WITH ALZHEIMER'S, CANCER, OR ANY DIAGNOSIS

the person they used to be. The writing is helpful and often humorous. What I truly enjoy is how the book not only gives guidance on how to improve the other person's life, but it also tells the reader how to appreciate their own time in life and how to enjoy it. One example is "So, choose carefully what you are giving your attention to. You are choosing your experience of life."

Having had a friend with Alzheimer's I can identify with much of what is said in this book. My only wish is that I had read it sooner before my friend passed away. David does an excellent job of letting the reader understand how to make the most of her time with her friend. I highly recommend this book to anyone with an older friend or relative who is facing the trials of dementia.

KATHY

❊ 🌿 ❊

I truly enjoy the book! The ideas are easy to understand and the book is the right length for me! Something I can read and apply right away. Some of the other books have been too long and overwhelming and I haven't even had the energy to tackle them. Thank you so much for thinking of my family! My dad has the book now.

RAE LYN

❊ 🌿 ❊

You have such a positive message, and your enthusiasm is infectious. I like your conversational tone and the use of the present tense (and your rationale for it.) Thanks for alternating the pronouns she and he. You inspire me!

KATHLEEN

❋ ⚘ ❋

My Mother has Alzheimer's. I want to let you know how much I appreciate your book "Live It Up!" I think I will carry it with me and re-read it when I need to.......but I want to say thank you for sharing this with me. I could connect very much with a lot of what you say and I will need this insight in the years to come. My Mother is in her early years of Alzheimer's, but the changes in her are still sometimes hard to deal with. Thank you for helping me to further understand.

ROSALIE

❋ ⚘ ❋

Dear David,

Thank you so much for your words of Wisdom and God's Love.

Sincerely,

ELLIE
(AN OLD GRANDMA)

❋ ⚘ ❋

LIVE IT UP!

SHARE A GREAT LIFE WITH ALZHEIMER'S, CANCER, OR ANY DIAGNOSIS

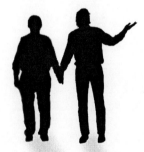

DAVID LAZAROFF

Live It Up! Share a Great Life With Alzheimer's, Cancer, or Any Diagnosis
Copyright © 2012 By David Lazaroff

Published by Expressionist Press LLC
Denver, Colorado
www.expressionistpress.com
877-926-9300

ISBN 13: 978-0-9851631-2-9

Printed in the United States of America.

DEDICATION

To
my wife, Meredith
who loves me through all my blunders

to
my mother
*who teaches me love is for
everyone, always*

to
my grandmother
*who teaches me what really
matters most*

to
Carl G. Carlson, Ph.D.
March 10, 1944 – January 21, 2011
I love you, my friend.

to
Gurumayi Chidvilasananda and
Swami Muktananda
You remind us we are all born in one love.

ACKNOWLEDGEMENTS

There are more people to acknowledge for their contribution to this book than I can possibly list. The fact is that I am who I am and this book is what it is due to every person I have come in contact with in my life. When a person comes in contact with another person, they impact and influence each other. Truly, we become each other. So, if you have interactions with me, your influence in my life is reflected in this book. The contributions of my friends, my family, my teachers, and my acquaintances throughout my life are reflected here. Even the people who grow the food I eat, stock the shelves at the store, and those who build my car and fuel it are reflected in the life I live, the words I write, and the people I serve. We all share the same world and by our presence, our words, and our actions, we become each other.

Still, there are a few who I acknowledge here by name: My mother Ann and my father Alan give me life and love that I share. My sisters Jacqueline, Suzanne, and Leslie share with me the joys of innocence and fun. My grandparents Eva, Sam, Elverda, and Lester who live on in the love of the families of their children. My wife Meredith who loves me in ways I am still learning to understand. My dear friend Carl Carlson whose life is given to the recognition of God in everyone and everything even so that his experience of Alzheimer's should offer others joy, love, and a beautiful experience of life, no matter what the health of their body or mind. My teacher Gurumayi Chidvilasananda and the lineage of teachers before her whose lives are given so that each of us might experience that we are born of a common love and we may share this world joyfully regardless of circumstances. Dr. Rudolph Ballentine who offers health and vitality as that which displaces disease and distress. Linda Bark, Ph.D. who gives her life so that others might experience their greatness. Tina, Mary, Megan, Joni, Di, Elizabeth, Annie, Kierre, Erika, Jack, Delmy, Jessica, Kevin, Jon, Vera, Holly, Abubakar, and Christine, whose care benefits Carl and others. Jonathan McCoy and Valerie McCoy who help elders with dementia complete their lives with love, dignity and lots of fun. Peggy Quinn, Rahima Dancy, and John Lainson. The people who I care for who demonstrate their willingness to experience joy regardless of the health of their body or mind: Rod, Helen, Masue, Harold, Edith, John, Ellen, Virginia, Sue, Pat, Betty, and Tap.

I acknowledge the contribution of the many people who I know from Landmark Education that believe in the abilities of all people. In particular, I thank Jeanine

Solomon, Sara Fabian, Jake Wilson, Rich Saalsaa, Juli Hall, Charlene Aframow, and Raemi Vermiglio. I thank all my fellow participants and coaches in the Landmark Education programs.

I acknowledge Kathleen Visovatti for her love and editing and being an example of living so others may have great lives. I thank Ardis Westwood who encourages me with her support and lives her life dedicated to spreading joy, love, and brotherhood. I thank Andrea Adler for more than I can list here.

I thank my writing coach, Kristen Moeller, for being a clearing in which this book is written. I thank the staff at Archer Ellison, Inc. who effectively brought this book from my computer into your hands.

CONTENTS

PREFACE

This book is written entirely in the present tense from my point of view. This is an odd way to speak continuously in the modern world. I break with conventions of relating to our history as past and that which has not happened as future. At times you may find speaking of history in the present tense requires sentence structures that are slightly unfamiliar. Please be patient as you become familiar with the unique rhythm of speaking entirely in the present tense. There are several reasons I do this.

First, this is how we really experience life: in the present moment, in the first person. We experience our food in the present, we experience our vision in the present, and we even experience our memories in the present. So, I do not dismember my memories and call them the past. I remember my history and live it again in the present. In this way I share my experience with you directly. In this way you, the reader, get to live my experience as your own. I find this more effective than telling you about my experience from a third person perspective as a past tense occurrence, distant to you and seemingly out of reach. I want you with me, experiencing the love, compassion, gentleness, and the choices I encounter in my life. I want you with me, experiencing my path of joy so you may more easily create your own path of joy with those you love.

Second, I am inspired to write in this way by the language and world view of the Hopi Indians of the American Southwest. Linguist Benjamin Lee Whorf (1897 – 1941) observes the Hopi language has "no words, grammatical forms, construction or expressions that refer directly to what we call `time.'" Can you stretch your mind to imagine time does not exist? Without a past or a future we have only one extending present moment. In such a view we have all that is called "past" and all that is called "future" in every moment. The present *is* the completion and result of the "past". The future *is* the completion and result of our present action. So, the future is not distinct from the present, rather it unfolds from within the present.

Third, as Alzheimer's advances, the cognitive ability to discern a past or future distinct and separate from the present diminishes. Notice it is a cognitive function to discern time and separate cause and effect. With the concept of time we say, "I push the glass off the table causing it to smash on the floor." Without the concept of time we say, "I push the glass off the table, smashing it on the floor." Holding cause and effect as separate is a higher cognitive function. Our present experience of life is with our attention, whether our attention is with music we are listening to or with a memory or with an imagined future. Holding your attention on "past" as distinct from "present" or "future" is a higher cognitive function. So, as Alzheimer's progresses and the higher cognitive functions wane, the person with Alzheimer's is left more and more entirely in the present moment, liberated from the concerns of the past and the future. In this way, for the person with advancing Alzheimer's related dementia, only that which holds attention is real, whether it is a memory, the weather, or a contrived thought or a distorted perception.

By attuning yourself to listen for the present experience of life, you are becoming more attuned to how the person with advancing Alzheimer's disease experiences the world. This prepares you to be present to their experience of the world, give your compassion, receive their love, and find the joy life is always offering.

Seeking out and discovering that which is not apparent is another higher cognitive function. As the friend of someone with Alzheimer's, you have this higher cognitive ability and you are able to seek out and find joy and bring it to the attention of your friend. By bringing joy to the attention of your friend and bringing your friend's attention to joy, you create a joyful experience of life in which you both can share.

The lessons of Alzheimer's apply to every state of human health. Why is this? When you strip away the higher cognitive functions and the layers of complexity and concealment these great mental capacities cover the basic human condition with, the fundamental needs of a human being are exposed. When these needs are exposed we can see what makes life an experience worth living. When we experience our access to the basic joys of life then we can embrace the greatness this life offers us and release that which is not consistent with the greatness. Thus the experience of a great life is available with any and every state of health!

INTRODUCTION

For a moment, please set aside all your experience with and knowledge about Alzheimer's disease, cancer, or any diagnosis you might greet with trepidation, fear, and sorrow. It is all valid. My purpose is to encourage you to explore the possibility of a new foundation for your concept of Alzheimer's and other diseases and what it means to you, your friends, and your loved ones. Later, you can retrieve what you know about these diseases and put it in place on top of the new foundation. Or, you can renew your pre-existing concepts, if that is more comfortable.

Life happens. People are born, and bodies grow quickly into a state of relative balance between the various organ and gland systems. After about 60 or 70 years organ systems, growing at different rates, move out of functioning in relative balance and eventually go into the completion of a sustainable balance. Many people call this *disease, old age,* or *dying.* Eventually the lungs and heart stop, the physical body dies and is buried, cremated or otherwise disposed of. A person's lifetime in the history of the Earth, is a very, very short time. Sometime along the way, the body may have opportunities to perpetuate the species by mating and reproducing.

The time from conception to completion of the physical life cycle, or living phase, of the *individual* human organism can vary from hours to months to years, or to decades. There are innumerable ways to influence the longevity of a body, but in the end, we all die.

The emotional life cycle of a human being is recognized as falling within the physical life cycle.

The spiritual life cycle of a human being is the subject of perpetual debate. Some say the spiritual life cycle completes within the confines of the physical life cycle. Some say the spiritual life cycle is bound to the life cycle of the species. Still others say the spiritual life cycle is continuous from the beginning of the Universe until its end.

This is all interesting, but it doesn't make much difference to most people. In this book I recognize variations from nominal operating balance of the systems of the physical body are only another context in which we make our emotional and spiritual journey. Alzheimer's and every other "disease" are ways in which the systems of the body are out of balance while the heart and lungs still function.

The existence of opportunities for joy, love, pleasure, companionship, and fulfillment is not diminished by the presence of Alzheimer's or any other "disease".

Joy is about what you like in life and that is available to you. What does it mean for something to be available or not available? Here is an example:

Carl loves to be the host at the meditation center. Being the host involves contemplating the monthly theme, researching scriptures and teachings on the theme, and preparing and delivering a ten-minute talk from his notes. These tasks involve cognitive abilities that are *available* to Carl. In other words, he has the cognitive ability at his command. He enjoys giving talks for many years. As Carl's Alzheimer's advances, Carl loses command of these mental abilities. The abilities to prepare sufficiently and deliver a ten-minute talk become *unavailable*.

Your experience of life is defined by where your attention is. As Carlos Castaneda says, "The trick is in what one emphasizes. We either make ourselves miserable, or we make ourselves happy." In every moment, life offers opportunities for sadness, disconnection, loneliness, regret, and sorrow. When our attention **lingers** on these, it is called suffering. Yes, there can be an end to suffering! The end of suffering involves moving our attention on to what we like and is available.

Life also offers, in every moment, opportunities for connection, love, play, companionship, and beauty. When our attention lingers on these, it is called happiness or joy.

So, choose carefully what you are giving your attention to. You are choosing your experience of life.

I am grateful for living seven years with the commitment my friend Carl, with a diagnosis of Alzheimer's, has a great life. My time with Carl is an experience of seeking and choosing joy.

I know Carl from a local meditation center. It is 2004 and I'm in my third year of attending programs at the center regularly. Carl is almost always smiling at the center. I know a bit of his history of losing his job as a psychologist in 2000 and not being able to hold a job since, and battling depression. On this day I find Carl outside the meditation hall after the morning program. His head hangs low in sadness.

"Carl, what's going on?" I ask.

Carl looks up at me with heavy and sullen eyes. "I'm gonna die." He says with resignation.

"Carl, we're all going to die. What's going on?"

Carl stammers, "I … I have Alzheimer's."

Finally, four years after losing his job, Carl has a diagnosis.

"Let's go for a walk," I suggest.

"OK."

We walk in the quiet shopping district under the warm sun.

"I don't know what I'm going to do. I don't have any money and I don't have any family."

I remember growing up and participating in the care of my grandparents as they age and complete their lives surrounded by family. They smile and find joy regardless of medical circumstances. I want Carl to have that same kind of love, care, and joy. I consider how my wife and I do not have children. We have considerable freedom with our time. My wife spends much time volunteering and I have a good job that affords me extra money. Carl is a generous person having given more than thirty years of devotion to his spiritual practices and care to thousands in his profession as a psychologist. I am considering giving my time and commitment to Carl. I have a persistent prayer in my life to serve others as part of my spiritual practices. All great spiritual traditions teach that to give selflessly and serve others with love is a path of great joy and rewards beyond imagination. I know I am setting the path for my life. It feels right to me. I make my next words as an offering to Carl, to my spiritual teacher, to God, and to all people who face disease, discomfort, fear, and loneliness:

"Carl, you have a life of service to others for more than thirty years through both your profession and through your spiritual practices. I want to be here for you. My wife and I don't have any kids. I have a good job. I can help you out. We can be buddies. Can I help you out?"

Carl pauses for a moment. "Why would you do this?" Carl asks.

"Our spiritual teacher, Gurumayi, wants us to have great lives. For thirty years you have meditation practices to quiet your mind. Now, your mind is going away of its own accord!" Carl does not appreciate my joke about his mind going away. I know appreciation for this might take years as the past and future wane and he is left with a present I make joyful.

"Okay, David. Thank you. You're a good friend."

Our lives are on a new course.

Here are a few simple principles that serve me well and are ready to serve you too.

Principle Number One: When you care for someone, fill their life with so much they like *and* is available to them, that there is no time left to dwell on desires for what is not available.

Principle Number Two: Apply Principle Number One to your own life so you have joy to give to your friend.

This book is a collection of vignettes offering perspectives on experiencing a great life and tangible ways you can share a great life when you, a friend or a relative has Alzheimer's, cancer, or another health condition. I invite you to be daring. Don't wait until disease is upon you or those you love. Take what you learn in this book and try it with everyone in your life, every day!

If you want support putting these practices into place in your professional practice or in your organization, I am available for coaching and training for individuals and organizations. I am also available for speaking.
Contact me: david@joyisavailable.com
877-926-9300

NEW PERSPECTIVES

Look for What You Like

If you like something and would like to have it in your life, then look for it. We find what we are looking for.

If you want to win a game, then play that game. We win games we play.

If you want to eat healthy foods, then buy healthy foods and fill your refrigerator with them. Eat your fill of healthy foods so there is no room for anything else.

If you are interested in cultivating happiness in your life, then think about the things that bring you happiness and act on them. When we put all our time on creating happiness, there is not room to linger on other things.

When you make your life about what you like that is possible, accessible, and available, then you are actively receiving what life is offering. When your mind strays from this, then your attention is nurturing something you do not like.

Look at the example of health. If you have a pulse, you have some degree of health. If you would like more health, focus on the areas of your life, your mind, and your body where you would enjoy more health. Explore more ways to increase your vibrancy and resiliency. Get help from experts who specialize in nourishing your organs that would benefit from nourishment and calming the organs that are more active than is beneficial. Good health is the result of nourishment and balance. A state of vibrant health is found in a pursuit of balance, not a battle for domination.

Mind your language and your thoughts. Preview your thoughts before you give them the power of your speech. Select the words that carry you to where you like to be. Do all your words support you in keeping focus on your goal? Keep the words that are useful and carry you forward. Release all others before you speak them.

I learn this from Carl. As Alzheimer's progresses, the abilities one often takes for granted recede and wane. When the abilities to read the newspaper or count money dissipate, it is time to look at what life is still offering and take it in so fully that the abilities of the past are left complete. Life is always offering joy, happiness, love, and fulfillment. If we are not experiencing these things, then we are not looking for them.

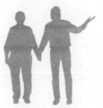

A New World

Watching the movie "A Beautiful Mind" I get a sense of how a person with dementia may experience the world differently than I do.

As I sit for meditation, my everyday way of experiencing the world dissolves and I emerge in an inner realm. It is a peaceful, steady world.

As Carl continues on his journey through life with Alzheimer's disease, his world changes as if he is moving from room to room in a funhouse at an amusement park: A room of mirrors, then a spongy floor, then walking through a spinning tube, darkness, a moving floor. Each room is its own world with its own perspective and laws of what is possible and what is appropriate.

Sitting with Carl, I look at him. "What world are you in now?" I wonder. I look in his eyes. He turns his head to gaze out the window. His eyebrows rise, a smile emerges and broadens. Carl chuckles. I follow his gaze to the squirrel clinging on the trunk of the tree, tail twitching. In this moment I enter Carl's world and I am with him completely. Life is good. We are fully present, together. My heart lifts in joy. I am present to the beauty of the squirrel's tail, softly filtering the light. I appreciate the curiosity, intensity and focus the squirrel is giving to its world; whatever is in its focus as it scurries up and down the tree. The agility is beautiful. The muscles ripple as the squirrel moves easily, sniffing at the bark. I am with Carl in a new world of beauty and companionship. I hold his hand as taught in Kindergarten. Life is offering beauty and we are receiving it.

Most of our lives are spent in our own inner world, in the solitude of our own perspective. A person can go on in relationships for years in their own worlds, assuming their friend or partner is sharing the inner experience, awakening one day to find he is the only audience to his soliloquy. I speak from experience.

What world are you in now? What is being offered to you? What is possible for you? Whose world do you dare enter? Whom do you invite into yours?

Thanks for the lesson, Carl.

How YOU Make a Difference

What does it really mean to make a difference? When you look at today and you look at yesterday, you can always see differences when you look for them. Life happens, even when we are not looking. We are on a course using resources and if we keep doing the same things every day, tomorrow holds a predictable picture of less resources, which certainly is different than today. So, an absolute difference between today and tomorrow is one kind of difference.

Another kind of difference we make is one that changes course and brings us to a destination different than what is predictable today. Sometimes the destination is not so predictable, but it is the possibility of a different path that excites our initiative.

There are differences of addition, subtraction, multiplication, and division. No, I'm not just talking about math. Some people are making a difference by signing petitions for funding for wildlife research (addition of money). Some people are raising their voices to stop whaling (subtraction of whale hunts). Others are advertising their causes in the mass media to multiply their support while many use language of fear and hate to divide perspectives and disperse their opponents.

I like the differences of transformation. As a transformative difference comes into being, the same circumstances take on a different meaning and present a new opportunity. One transformational difference I am making is how we, in the United States, relate to the events of growing old until our body ceases to function. Today this is called "dying". I am making this transform into "completing one's life". This is a big difference. It will take time and effort to make it. There is a great difference in the experience of the event if one relates to it as death or one relates to it as completion. How one relates to the event impacts how one cares for the being going through the event. The choice of words has tremendous power for us. Would you rather die? or would you rather complete your life? How does your perspective shape how you live today?

What is your mode of making a difference? When you are making your difference, however you choose to go about it, please do it with intention and passion so when your time comes to complete your life, you know you have expressed yourself fully and you are complete with your life.

I offer personal and organizational coaching and consulting in creating transformational change. If you want support in transformation, contact David Lazaroff:
http://www.joyisavailable.com/coaching
877-926-9300

All the Time In the World

Hey! What's the rush? You have all the time in the world. Are you forgetting this?

No kidding, you have 24 hours every day. There is no more time in the whole world (with the exception of sub-atomic particles that experience time dilation at relativistic speeds, but let's not go there). So, what's your hurry?

One day in 2004 my friend Carl shows me a quote from his spiritual teacher, Swami Muktananda: "Time eats all things. But God eats time. He eats time like chutney." Carl laughs so heartily at the quote, he can hardly speak.

Recently, after years of rolling around in my head, this quote blossoms and I reach a new understanding of what Muktananda tells us. Muktananda also teaches, "God dwells within you, as you." So, I see we are the time-eaters. We get all the time in the world: each and every one of us gets 24 hours per day. Like one who puts chutney, or ketchup, or salsa, or jam on their food to add flavor, we put time on the activities of our life and make those activities where we put time, richer, and enhanced.

On what are you putting your time? Study, love, play? Look at what you have in life. It is nourished by you with the water of time. If you put your time to other things, they will grow in your life.

Carl can no longer speak as he did six years ago. He has Alzheimer's disease and the course of time has taken away much of the control of his physical and mental functions. But, Carl has peace because he cultivated it with his life of kindness and spiritual practices. Not even time with Alzheimer's has been able to take this away from him.

What are you cultivating today? Your own tomorrow. You have all the time in the world.

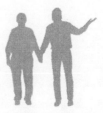

A Present For You

This present is for you. This is ALL there is.

I am happy you are here NOW. I am happy to be here with you.

Please enjoy this present. Recall the love in your life. Recall your friends. Recall all the people in your life whose contributions make this present just what it is: everything you create with your life.

Open your heart and let it be filled with this present. Open your hands and your arms and embrace only this present.

It is only in this present you experience your history. It is only in this present your life unfolds.

All joy is available in this present. Do you see the joy? Are you finding the joy? Look again. Look persistently. Focus your mind on this present. Be still. This is your life. This is all there is. Choose the joy. Meditate on the joy. Meditate on the beauty.

Now... look around... see the joy everywhere!

The Life I Love

Oooooo… I have chills just thinking about it: The life I love. Where is it? Oh, it's HERE!

Everything I enjoy is at hand. My guitar, a good paying job, my wife, my sisters and parents are just a phone call away, friends I love, health, exercise, yoga, meditation, sunny days, nature, inner peace. Yet, sometimes I forget.

Forgetfulness: a trick of the mind; the mind astray. The moments I stop seeing the things I love that are all around me are the moments I feel disconnected and lonely. Then I am distracted…. I'm off to my "bad habits" and a few hours of wasted time my intellect and self-image can't quite get a grip around, which leaves me with a feeling of guilt and disconnectedness. Or it can last days, weeks, or months. Yes, disconnected amidst all the things I can identify as important, vital, and fulfilling to me.

There's a hole in my life and I can hear the echo of its depths, but I can't see it. It's in a blind spot. Hey! Those distractions are telling me something. Those wandering thoughts are clues. There's something missing, the presence of which would make a difference: passion in my personal relationships… freely expressing my care and joy for the company of others… my joy for you.

I love you. Yes, you. Now that I can say it, now that I can see it, now that I can feel it freely and simply, my life is a more joyful experience. I'm connected, again. I can focus on my guitar practice, composing, relationships, job, exercise, yoga, meditation, sunny days, health, nature, and be present to the inner peace that is always present, waiting for my attention.

What's your distraction? What is it telling you? What's missing in your way of being, the presence of which would make a difference? The world has everything we love and all the ingredients to the life we want to live are available. Can you hear the clues that will reveal the blind spots?

If you want a transformation around experiencing more joy in your life, I recommend the Landmark Forum: http://www.landmarkforum.com I also offer personal and organizational coaching. Contact David Lazaroff: http://www.joyisavailable.com/coaching 877-926-9300

This Year Has Everything You Want in Life

This year has everything you want in life. Are you ready to receive it? The happiness and joy? Go for it! When you declare it, it is so. When you are looking for the happiness life is offering you, you can see it, feel it, even swim in it. Can you keep your eye on it? Can you pursue what you really want? Of course you can! Do you have the will to stick to it? Are you following your heart's beat for joy?

I invite you on a journey through the happiest year in your life. Are you with me? Now, let's be clear what we are in for. This year will be the happiest, because you say so and because you are actively tuning-in to and responding to the joy life is offering you more than you have any other year. Truly, happiness and joy are around you as much as the air you breathe. Oh, you don't notice the air you are breathing? Luckily your lungs know how to pluck the oxygen out and leave the nitrogen and other gasses for your exhale. You do this so effortlessly, so, you can think about other things… like how life is offering you joy every minute. Together, let's try to train our minds to pluck the joy from life around us at all times.

Today I am in pursuit of how I am connected to the people around me. So, this morning I'm out clearing my sidewalk of snow. I notice the neighbor who has an at-home daycare hasn't been home to shovel her walk. The snow is dry, light, and the shoveling is easy. I clear my sidewalk to her property line and continue to clear her walk. I recognize how she always greets me with a smile and teaches children how to have fun and get along. She does not know I am shoveling. I see her smile in my heart.

What joy are you finding today?

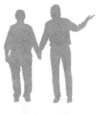

Do What You Really Want To Do

I have a lot of things I can do. You have many things you can do. We have choices… lots of choices.

This morning I have some of my favorite distractions calling me. I have my music calling me. I have my meditation practice calling me. Reading, learning, blogging, etc. Honestly, no matter my choice, nobody dies. Do you recognize all the choices you have every minute? I look at all the expectations I put on my life yesterday and yesterdays before that. Those expectations I lay for myself really don't matter as much as I think when I create them. I'm a different person now.

I reach for the life I want to live today. I see life newly today. I dismiss the distractions and choose to dive into my life with my meditation.

I sit in my meditation room noticing how breathing deeply moves my body into alignment. My mind chatter subsides, returns, and subsides again. I find the quiet point in my chest, in my heart. My muscles relax. Each full inhalation expands my ribs to the front and sides, removing the slump from my exhalation and supporting my spine in an erect, natural curve.

I have lots of things to choose from. I choose to fully enjoy this stillness. I am re-energized, at peace, and grateful. My mind chimes in reminding me this is going very well and I've done a good job at following my meditation teacher's first instruction: "Take a comfortable posture." My cushion is firm. My legs are supported. I relax completely with comfort.

Ten minutes pass and I hear my wife pull into the driveway. I choose to spend some time with her. Reading and blogging is available later.

Are you choosing your activities with joy? Do you use the full power of your choice to create your happiness?

Do your best to have a great life with your friends and family in every circumstance. If you want help in seeing the great life around you, try getting a coach. I am available for coaching:
David Lazaroff
http://www.joyisavailable.com/coaching
877-926-9300

Double Rainbow

I accelerate onto I-25 for my 20 minute morning commute to work. I'm in the sun and there are dark skies to the West. WOW! A double rainbow like none I've ever seen before! The morning sun illumines the coming storm; the ends of the main arch radiate disproportionately.

A rainbow is the perception of the colorful refraction of light off of water in the air. A rainbow is seen from a distance. You can never touch a rainbow.

Rainbows have such meaning in various cultures. The Irish legends of gold at the end of a rainbow are testaments to the gullibility of people who would chase after something that can only be perceived at a distance. I reflect on my own dreams I chase in life and wonder if I am just chasing for a pot of gold at the end of a rainbow, being gullible.

Then there is the biblical story of Noah and his ark. As the great flood finally recedes, the ark comes upon dry ground. God makes his covenant; such a flood will never destroy all creatures again. The bow in the clouds is forever to be the sign of the covenant. I am warmed by this story given to me as my heritage. I am heartened the Divine is present in my life and visible on this morning.

Yes, the rainbow can only be perceived from a distance. Yet, the perception of a rainbow shows us the full spectrum of light is with all sunlight everywhere. Similarly, life is full of divine experiences and miracles. Sometimes we are too close to these experiences to perceive the miraculous. Saints do not perceive the miraculous in their actions: a saint is recognized as a saint by those who observe their deeds and outcomes from afar.

Of course, I can make anything or nothing of my encounter with this rainbow. The center of the arch is directly ahead of me, between me and the Rocky Mountains. I feel like I am heading into a portal to a heavenly realm.

But enough of this other-worldliness. I can make today a heavenly experience of joy, peace, and love. Yes, the center of this rainbow may very well be my office at the Denver Federal Center in Lakewood. What will I make of today? It is off to a good start, and I have my guitar in the back of my car for a visit with Carl this evening.

Accepting the rainbow as a sign of God's love, I experience beauty in the world and a connection with others. I appreciate the love in others. I feel stronger, braver, and at peace. Life really is what we make of it. I choose this life and this experience.

What do you choose today?

Gratitude

Gratitude refreshes and gives life. Do you feel it? Gratitude scatters the shadow of loneliness with the light of recognition of the contribution others are to who we are. And to be fair and complete, gratitude is the recognition of our importance to others, that they think enough of us to give something we are grateful for.

When I am grateful for you, I hold you in my heart. When I remember you, I am uplifted. In a moment, the world appears whole, friendly, and joyful. I am communing with a friend, recognizing love. I am free to hold hands, smile, jump, and dance. Laughter sends from my belly through my lungs and out my mouth, tickling me with life.

I am comforted remembering you are only a thought away. You welcome my call and I welcome yours. Without ever seeing you, I know it is by our lives, collectively, that the world offers us what is possible.

I am grateful for your kindness, your compassion, your smile, your laughter, your intensity, your ease, your love. I am grateful for your curiosity, your humanity, your humility, your generosity, your tenacity. I am grateful for your wit, your friendliness, your playfulness, your timeliness, your beauty, your health, and your strength. You have all these things in the proportions adding up to YOU! For all this, I am grateful for you. This is who you are for me.

For you, I wish only the best. My joy is to see you express your qualities, expanding your contribution, and engaging with the qualities of others, sated every day with companionship and self-recognition for the contribution you are.

I am grateful for you. Thank you.

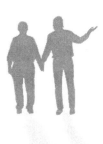

The Beauty of Caring

Key to World Peace Found
With Elderly and Frail

As Carl's friend, companion and advocate, over a six year period, I learn many lessons about disability insurance, elder law, assisted living, and what people care about. But Carl's eyes teach me the most profound lessons. As operating a washing machine becomes too complex, we discover the joy of meeting with the owner of the laundry service twice weekly. Carl laughs at this man's broad Philippine smile and the proprietor laughs at how many pairs of socks and underwear Carl brings in, many only having been taken out of last week's cleaning and thrown on the floor because of a wrinkle not to Carl's liking.

As Carl's speech becomes simpler, I learn of his love of music and with him I attend dozens of concerts, until the stairs and crowds become unworkable. Every time an ability recedes I look to find what life is offering that is workable and enjoyable. Life is always offering adventure and joy. We can always find them when we look for them. Carl teaches me the power of raising an eyebrow and sporting a half-cocked grin is more precise communication than any lengthy explanation... as long as I'm paying attention.

Carl reveals, by example, what ancient sages tell us: when we are living in the present moment, we find peace. This is perhaps the biggest lesson. As Carl's Alzheimer's advances, his experience of life shifts more easily with his internal state and external stimuli. Some senses are magnified and others are filtered. The means to communicate with him is to become completely present to his world, enter it, and experience what is of greatest importance to him in the moment. This is attending to his needs, recognizing his humanity, becoming his companion again and again, and creating the space for his love, appreciation, and other offerings to express.

When we practice this with our elders, we can bring this skill to our neighbors and when we can do this with our neighbors, we have more access to interacting with other cultures and nations in this way. This is an access to peace. Peace begins with each of us, with you.

I am committed to people experiencing love and joy in the caring process. To help you , I have resources listed in the back of this book. I am also available for consulting in support of you and those you care for.
Contact David Lazaroff
http://www.joyisavailable.com/coaching
877-926-9300

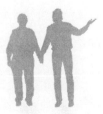

The Upward Spiral of Joy

Today has everything the world offers. Look no further for your next action or your next joy. The door to the world of joy is open today.

Beware expectations of the future. We have only today. Today the world turns. Today the world turns. What is a day? Why slice up your life. We have only this breath, this breath, this breath.

Collect the joy of today into your heart. The future you imagine arises from today only. Look around for the beauty and love today offers you. Yes, today offers you non-joy AND today offers you JOY! What are you filling your mind with? What are you filling your heart with? Choose your filling! What will it be? Sadness, mediocrity, or joy? I recommend the joy with a generous topping of love.

Carl's Alzheimer's is progressing. Carl looks at me, confused as to how he should feel. He seems to notice what busy minds miss: he's never had this moment before. However I am being, Carl mirrors me with magnification. If I am sad, Carl is sullen. If I am happy, Carl is giddy. When I am with him, I am his world. Truly, I am creating his world for him! I notice this, so I make an effort to fill myself with love and joy. I pay attention to be clear in my communication with my wife so I can carry happiness from my marriage with me into my visits with Carl.

You have the experience of others creating your world for you. Do you recall being in a meeting or other gathering when someone walks into the room bringing their anger, cynicism, and hostility? The mood of everyone in the room is immediately brought into the shadow of resignation, withdrawal, and trepidation. In a moment your world is recreated by the presence of another.

Or, there is a prevailing sense of glumness in a room and a joyful and warm person walks in with their smile beaming. The newcomer is established in their joy and steadfast in their disposition. The joy spreads as smiles resonate to all present and moods are lifted.

In my time with Carl, I discover an upward spiral of joy. If I show up with joy and love in my heart, Carl begins to reflect it back, making me more at ease and happier still. If I am forgiving with him, he finds comfort in my presence making me aware my efforts bear fruit in his peace. Each smile from one person brings forth a greater smile reflecting from the other. The joy moves from sublime to subtle to visible to audible!

For me the choice to create joy is like walking into the house of life with a stairway down into the dark basement and another to the patio on the roof under the open sky and sunshine. We always have this choice. I like the view from the roof. It is more work to climb the stairs, but this is where the joy is.

Be at peace with today. Create an upward spiral of joy!

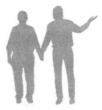

Joy: The Antidote to Misery and Suffering

To pursue joy is not to whitewash the challenges and sadness of life. Sadness, fear, and challenges are very real experiences. These experiences distract us from the joys of life and it is critical to the happiness of everyone to complete them and move through them appropriately and NOT GET STUCK. We see supporting examples of this in many cultures around rituals and practices of burial and grieving. There is an appropriate (although not precisely fixed) time for grief and an appropriate time to move beyond grief.

There is a distinction between validating an experience of fear and validating that which is feared. Here is an example from my past: When caring for Carl through the early stages of Alzheimer's, I have a valid experience of fear of handling his care when the time comes when he is incontinent. I know this time is coming. I'm grossed out by the thought of it.

I reflect back on my childhood when grandma uses a commode and later a bed pan as her strength withers from cancer. Mom assists grandma with all her hygiene. Mom always has a look of sincere care and love in her eyes. Her every movement expresses her compassion.

I am peering with fear into a future that has not

yet happened and might never happen. I don't even realize I'm making it all up in my head: "Will he let me help him? What if he is combative?"

However, I do not need to validate incontinence as being fearsome. Doing so only impedes my ability to move through my experience of fear and prepare myself to handle assisting Carl with toileting and incontinence. In truth, incontinence is not fearsome, it is just human hygiene. It is also true it is valid and common for people to have a fear of assisting the incontinent when they have no experience doing so.

So, at this time of fear I look for what is joyful: Carl is my friend. He trusts me to care for him. Making sure he is clean and comfortable is one way to express my love for him and give him a good life. When I help him use the toilet at a concert hall, we can comfortably get back to our seats and enjoy the music. When I help him in the family restroom at the stadium, we can get back to enjoying the ball game in comfort.

In this way, looking for joy helps us acknowledge, complete, and move through times of fear, sadness, and loss. It is OK to experience these feelings. It is not OK to be stuck there, bear with it, and just get through a miserable day to recreate the misery tomorrow. That is a life of suffering and I insist we interrupt suffering with joy. The alternative is unimpeded and uninterrupted suffering. I'm not OK with that, are you?

I stand for people having joyful lives in any and every circumstance. Will you join me? What do you stand for?

Find your joy!

Do you need help finding your joy? I'm here for you! Look into the resources at the back of this book or contact me:
David Lazaroff
http://www.joyisavailable.com/coaching
877-926-9300

Cure for All Suffering Found!

Do you notice that when you are full with joy, there is no room for sadness or suffering? I learn this, as a child, from my grandmother as she progresses through colon cancer. Grandma moans in pain. My mother comes to her side. "Mom, would you like some morphine for the pain?"

Grandma declines, "I want my mind clear, I want to see my grandchildren." When she is with her family, regardless of the pain, grandma is not suffering, she is enjoying life.

More than thirty five years later, I am still appreciating the depths of lessons from Grandma. I recognize the same lessons coming from others. Carl continues to teach me since 2004 when the doctor gives him a diagnosis of Alzheimer's Disease and I begin helping him. As dementia progresses, frustration swells from time to time. These are moments of suffering, like a dream of running for your life, but not getting anywhere, except it is real.

Suffering is the experience of our attention lingering on a subject in a state of despair. A frightening or frustrating experience is not suffering. A painful experience is not suffering. Keeping our attention in a state of despair on a frightening, frustrating, or painful experience is suffering. Suffering is when we cling to distress and focus on that which we do not like or that which we desire and is not available.

Grandma's lessons teach me how to cure Carl's suffering. I hold his hand and look into his eyes. I smile and let him know love is with him and I value him for the love he gives as he squeezes my hand. I play guitar and sing to him. I walk with him in the park. He still has memory loss and dementia, but he is joyful and his suffering is cured. When a new suffering arises, Carl's caregivers know how to cure that one too.

Compassionate companionship displaces suffering. Take the time to hold hands, look into eyes, and enter the world of another. You can displace suffering with love and a sense of ease, regardless of the physical circumstances. Engaged loving care is the cure for suffering. Try adding it on top of your current medical plan! No prescription necessary. No negative side-effects. Apply liberally, as needed. Unlimited refills.

Note that when choosing to accept or decline medication, my Grandma is lucid and mentally competent to make such a choice. Choices to administer or withhold medications should be taken with consideration to the patient's preference. When the patient is not mentally competent, the person with medical powers of attorney should consult with physicians and legal experts when making a choice regarding the administration of medications.

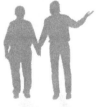

The Glory of Friendship

Glory – Great beauty or splendor, that is so overwhelming it is considered powerful.

Your friend is feeling down, so you visit to lift her spirits. You give your friend a gift and she is emotionally moved. You laugh with her every chance you get. Your friend asks you to help achieve something very important to her, and you help if you can. Your friends are a great source of beauty and power in your life. You trust them, you will do anything they ask.

Do you notice how much your friends are there for you? They see you as a gift to their life. They're glad when you ask them to join you in your hobbies, your play, or what you believe in. Even if they decline your invitation, they are glad you think enough of them to ask. So, if you find a cause you believe in and are supporting, tell your friends. If you want to see something happen and you are working for it, tell your friends what it means to you.

I have countless hours with Carl over the six years since his Alzheimer's diagnosis. I help because Carl has a life of being there for others and because I benefit from his efforts to help open the meditation center I attend. I do it because I want someone to be there for me and I want people to have the kind of loving care given to my grandparents. The net result is a lot of emotional and spiritual benefit for me, the most poignant being when Carl looks at me piercingly and says, "You're a good friend."

Being a good friend is the very best thing you can do for yourself and for your friends. With a friend, loneliness is dispersed, pain is dulled, and angst is eased. Joy is cultivated inside of friendship. The act of giving to a friend is quickly self-rewarding.

I suggest taking some time to offer friendship to someone for whom it makes a great difference. Visit a nursing home or assisted living home. Adopt an elder, offer companionship, lend an ear and listen. Share yourself and allow them to be your friend.

Experience the glory of friendship.

Friendship – the Vehicle of Joy

What can make the difference in caring for someone with Alzheimer's or another disease?

Friendship.

When caregivers and those with Alzheimer's are friends, they are watching out for each other. A friend does not miss an upset and can enter your world in a moment and hold your hand and lead you through any darkness into a smile. Love between friends is palpable. There is no loneliness in friendship. When you are with your friend and you are in your friendship, joy is available! Circumstances do not matter. A friend does not turn their back when you are in need. A friend has time. A friend listens closely to both verbal and non-verbal communication, knows what you like and what makes you laugh and uses this knowledge to lift your spirits. A friend delights in your presence, appreciates your every breath and tells you.

Am I suggesting every relative, caregiver, social worker, and staff person in a home caring for someone with Alzheimer's should be committed to the person with Alzheimer's as a lifelong friend? Yes. This environment cannot fail to produce a joyful life for all. While this does not remove the medical condition, it cures the dis-ease. When every dollar spent on Alzheimer's produces a smile on the face of a patient, family member, caregiver, or friend, then Alzheimer's will be welcomed as a wellspring of joy. Let's put the money where the joy is.

When someone loses the past, give them a present of love and joy. Do not rob their present with sadness, remorse, and pining for disappointments of plans for a future that never was and will never be. Share love NOW. There is no other time.

I am committed that persons with long term illnesses and those nearing the completion of their lives have the opportunity to experience joy in their circumstance. If you or your organization want support in experiencing this kind of joy, contact me:
David Lazaroff
http://www.joyisavailable.com/coaching
877-926-9300

Joy: The Primary Focus of Care

I assert: love, joy, and companionship are the fundamental requirements of health care. Any other care that may be regulated and enforced to ensure physical health and safety should be delivered in the context of ensuring the presence of love, joy, and compassion. If the delivery of food, shelter, medicine, hygiene, and other physical care is made in the absence of love, joy, and companionship in the experience of the receiver, then the delivery is inadequate.

Physical suffering is obvious to a third party and therefore easy to regulate and intervene upon by an observer. Mental and emotional health are less obvious and require much more attention to discern and attend to. Spiritual health is still more subtle. The cultivation of understanding of the mental and emotional health of another person is accomplished in the context of personal relationships over time. Particularly skillful and sensitive persons can sometimes gain insights to the joy and suffering of an individual quickly, but time and relationship must be respected as the primary sources of authority. Spouses, family members, and caregivers with long-standing relationships and observable commitment to a person receiving care can create a mentally and emotionally safe environment that overrides some apparent physical hazards or threats.

Great considerations deserve attention when removing a person from their mentally and emotionally safe environment to provide a more physically safe environment. If the provision of a physically safer environment causes enduring mental and emotional misery, a great assault on the person's humanity occurs. The person with dementia is often unconcerned and unaware of their physical condition and their world perception is in the mental and emotional realm. With Alzheimer's related dementia present, Maslow's hierarchy is askew as the sense of love and belonging is a more basic need than physical safety. In this context, without love and belonging, a physically sustaining environment is a prison of loneliness, sorrow, and grief with no hope for parole.

An article on Chill4Us.com explores the question "What good is it making someone safer if it merely makes them miserable?" (http://chill4us.com/news/what-good-is-it-making-someone-safer-if-it-merely-makes-them-miserable%25e2%2580%2599) as a legal inquiry. The crux of the problem is in the headline, which implies misery is unrelated to safety. This is a false premise. Misery is a threat to the safety of basic measures of health in the human condition: peace, love, and a sense of belonging. To introduce misery is to threaten these securities. Misery is an unsafe condition.

In the physical human form we experience the mental, emotional, and spiritual worlds through the relationships we develop with others and the physical world. The only proper context for physical care is in support of a **JOYFUL** mental, emotional, and spiritual experience.

If you are a health care professional and you want to help your patients live more joyful lives, or if you work in a long term care facility and you want your residents to have a more joyful experience every day, call me and I will help you achieve your goal:
David Lazaroff
http://www.joyisavailable.com/coaching
877-926-9300

Hiring Friendship in a Care Home

Are you happy with all the caregivers at a facility where a loved one lives?

The job descriptions of caregivers do not say "friend". So, don't expect it. Their performance is not evaluated on their friendship. So, don't expect it. The structures of the homes and the evaluation of performance of managers and administrators do not emphasize friendship. So, don't expect it. This is unrealistic.

It is more natural for a person to befriend and love another person than it is for them to put on a uniform and go to a job for a shift of 8, 10, 12, 24, or 72 hours to keep records, follow procedures, be mindful of regulations, and tend to whatever pleases their supervisor. It is unrealistic to think it is more difficult and takes more time to train a person to be loving and compassionate than it takes to train them to bathe, dress, transfer, feed, and assist another person in the use of a toilet. People who are suitable to care for the elderly and frail have experienced friendship, joy, love, and companionship for many more years than any formal training in policies, procedures, and regulations.

Why are people with Alzheimer's and other conditions of frailty dying of boredom, loneliness, and helplessness in beautiful homes staffed by capable, "well trained," compassionate people? Because, it is UNREALISTIC to expect joy and companionship to flourish where the center of efforts is on business structures and regulations.

Only when the joy, love, and companionship of those being cared for are the measures of effectiveness and success of caregivers, staff, and administrators does the opportunity for joyful living and a comforting completion of life become fully realized. When a caregiver is asked, "What do you do for a living?" the response should be, "I love people."

How do you do this if you are running a care home? You begin by putting love and concern for the joy of your residents and staff (yes, staff) first. Only joyful staff can cultivate joy for residents. Then put joy and friendship first in the job descriptions. You must expect it and participate in it. Pay the staff well and give them shifts that leave them energy for their families. Train them to first attend to the joyful experience of those they care for.

I am committed to making a joy filled life available to people in all circumstances. I have done it and I know what it takes. What are you committed to?

If you operate an assisted living home or nursing care facility and you find it difficult to create effective policies that support nurturing friendships between staff and residents, I can help you. Contact:
David Lazaroff
http://www.joyisavailable.com/coaching
877-926-9300

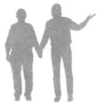

The Purpose of Life is Found in Caring

An editorial in The Florida Times-Union (http://jacksonville.com/opinion/editorials/2011-10-16/story/hidden-disease-needs-our-attention October 15, 2011) warns the US is on a track to spend $20 trillion on Alzheimer's care in the next 40 years. One in eight people who live beyond age 65 will be diagnosed with dementia before their life is complete. Special "memory care" units charge $7,000 per month or more. Alzheimer's is a one way road for the body. There is no recovery or cure. Are there solutions to this problem?

Yes, there are solutions. These require new thinking. The thinking that memory care needs to cost $84,000 per year is broken. The lack of strong medical models for intervention, prevention and cure, call for sustainable care models.

The solution resides in our neighborhoods and families. Keep in mind you have a place in these statistics! The one-in-eight mentioned who will develop Alzheimer's includes your parents, your siblings, your friends, your neighbors, and YOU! Are you the one diagnosed or among the seven friends and family members?

So, let's make it personal and assume YOU have the diagnosis. As your cognitive abilities decline, how are your emotional and spiritual health be cared for? How do you avail yourself of the beauty and joy the world still offers? Who do you want near you? Whose face brings you comfort? Whose touch makes you feel alive? What music will makes your spirit dance?

You live in a place you love, don't you? Isn't this why you moved into your neighborhood? Do you have friends or family in your neighborhood? Do you belong to a religious organization or service club in your neighborhood? Do you know the people you see at the grocery store or hardware store or park or bus stop? If the answer to all of these is "no", then consider enjoying your neighborhood more or moving to someplace you can enjoy.

The current model of $84,000 per year care is based upon moving you away from your neighborhood to a place where strangers will attend to what needs they can until you are dead. It may be a difficult long journey for your friends and loved ones to visit, so visits are infrequent. There's not a budget to get you to your Rotary Club meetings where you've had lunch on Tuesdays for the last 30 years, so you have to make due with whatever appears from the mysterious kitchen and an activity designed for people like you. The problem is you are not like other people and your *friends and family* know what you respond to on levels beyond cognition.

In a small neighborhood assisted living home, it costs about $100 per day or $36,500 per year to care for a person who is not well enough to live on their own. Every neighborhood should have such a home. This cost level is achieved at a home with 10 to 12 residents when there is a mixture of residents with and without cognitive impairments and physical impairments. Concentrating and segregating persons with Alzheimer's degrades YOUR quality of life, drives up costs, and isolates you from the life you have created for decades.

A solution involves creating a home in your neighborhood where you can go to complete your life when living in your home becomes unworkable. The solution involves you participating in caring for your family member, friend, and neighbor while you are still able and receiving the care of others when you need to.

Your "primary caregiver" needs support and you need the support of more than one person. It is a lot of hard work to keep joy afloat in your life and it is the most rewarding work! Before your cognition declines too far, organize your friends and family with lotsahelpinghands.com so many people can share the effort of helping you complete your life in a loving, dignified and enjoyable way.

Caring for others is not a burden and distraction from the opportunities of life. Caring for others, and being cared for, is the POINT of life. Yes, I am revealing to you the meaning of life! Remember: when we share the load, we can carry any weight. When we share the work, we can build a structure of any size or a road of any length. To ignore life's opportunity to live and complete life in community is to be ignorant of the source of joy and happiness in the world.

The frailty accompanying the completion of life is our invitation to participate fully in life. When we engage in this process as a community, it is enriching. When we outsource love and care, it is very, very expensive.

Are you creating long-term care solutions that are more effective and less expensive? If you want help in identifying the factors that make life great for people caring and people being cared for, I'm here to help. Contact:
David Lazaroff
http://www.joyisavailable.com/consulting
877-926-9300

Beyond Coping: Having a Great Life!

Pam LeBlanc writes on Austin360.com: "Exercise helps patients cope with Alzheimer's Disease" (http://www.austin360.com/recreation/exercise-helps-patients-cope-with-alzheimers-disease-1889621.html Pam LeBanc, Oct. 1, 2011). Pam gives the example of John Duncan, a man with Alzheimer's who enjoys life more with regular personal training than he did before personal training. The personal training experience gives him better strength, balance, mobility, and cognitive function. To add to Pam's article, I want to point out the depth of the impact the personal training experience has on persons with Alzheimer's such as John Duncan. The impact goes far beyond "coping". The lesson presented also has a scope that goes far beyond Alzheimer's. This is a lesson for everyone to imbibe with any level of health. When a person is having a good time exercising, listening to music, making love, or simply holding hands, they are having a joyful life.

The word "coping" implies a contextual background of struggle, loss, or unfortunate circumstances. Seeing a "background", for the context of an activity or how an activity occurs for a participant, is a higher cognitive function. Being aware of a context or background requires holding the past and future in mind at the same time with the present focus of attention. As Alzheimer's progresses, background and context disappear as the mind only holds the present experience. Even if it is a memory that is the focus of the moment, the particular memory is experienced in the present without an additional context.

For John Duncan, training is its own enjoyable experience. During the workout, he is only present to his participation and is not concerned with whether or not he has Alzheimer's, what he will do tomorrow, or what he used to have for a profession. His experience is not one of coping, but one of enjoyment of movement, fitness, nature, and the companionship of his personal trainer. He is free of worry and engaging in a workout in a way worthy of the aspirations of the most cognitively sound persons. John is well cared for. While enjoying his workout, John is having a great life!

There is a valuable lesson here for people of high cognitive function: Be willing to give up your construct of a past and future that is independent and separate from the present. Enjoy what life is presenting to you for enjoyment NOW! Consider that the joys of life are most deserving of your attention and that the non-joy of life is a distraction from the joy that is immediately available. Consider that although you are experiencing pain or sorrows or disconnection, joy is available right in front of you. Perhaps the joy is in a blind spot, obscured by circumstances or the tendency of your mind to linger on what you now find unpleasant? Perhaps the joy is calling for you to take action in order for you to become present to it?

Yes, exercise can improve the functions of the body, including the brain. But, the real lesson here is: the goal of therapies and interventions deserves to go beyond coping, relieving symptoms, and restoring function. Sometimes restoration is something that will not happen. The true goal is to have a great life, enjoying all life offers that is available for enjoyment.

*If you want to train caregiving staff to be present
to the impact they have on the lives of their
patients, I can provide that training. Contact:
David Lazaroff
http://www.joyisavailable.com/consulting
877-926-9300*

10 Ways to Share Joy When Your Friend Has Alzheimer's

Share Humor

Humor invokes a joyful state. You might have a history of fun and laughing with your friend. Your history with your friend might be one of a work environment with few intimate laughing moments. Either way, be assured this humor is available!

Your friend's sense of humor may change on her path through Alzheimer's. So, approach humor as an ongoing inquiry or exploration. As you spend time with your friend, notice what she laughs about. Notice what she complains about, what she finds absurd, and what she finds silly. Notice what provokes smirks, smiles, giggles, and laughter that stops only when she's too tired to continue laughing.

When your friend finds humor, enter her world and join in the fun. Your friend is happy when laughing alone. When you join in the joy, it becomes a party!

Humor comes in many forms including jokes, puns, and riddles. When you recall past sources of laughter for your friend, try them out again. Celebrate with a good laugh if it makes your friend laugh. If she doesn't get it, move on to something else.

Humor is intimate and personal. Be willing to enter your friend's world and play from within her perspective. If sharing in your friend's sense of humor is not working for you, just try sharing in her joyful state simply for the reward of the laughter. You can experience joy for its own sake, separate from humor. To say it simply: If your friend finds something funny and you don't get it, humor her and join in the laughter.

❋ ⚘ ❋

I'm on a drive with Carl to go to a movie. Suddenly, Carl perks up, his eyes widen in surprise and joy. His jaw drops open, and he starts jabbing his finger in the air, pointing out into the traffic. "Hey! Hey! Hey!"

I'm getting alarmed! "What? What?" My eyes dart between Carl, his finger, and the traffic where he is pointing.

Carl laughs heartily in astonishment, "Crunch!!," he calls out.

My confusion clears when I finally see it: There is a sedan driving in the lane to our left, just a few yards ahead. The bumper is missing and the right, rear quarter panel is dented and folded. I look to Carl mirroring his excitement, "That car?"

"Yeah," he exclaims, and belts out a hearty laugh, slapping his knee with joy.

I get it! Carl likes things neat and in order. If something is broken, he likes to get it fixed. If I have a thread or fuzz on my shirt, Carl notices it and picks it off for me with a smile. When he sees a damaged car driving down the street with all the nice cars, he can't contain his laughter at such an out of place sight.

From this point on, every dented or dirty car rewards our attention with a good laugh from Carl. Carl laughs and I laugh out of the joy of sharing in Carl's happiness.

Hold Hands

We learn to hold hands in kindergarten. Then we grow up and reserve hand holding for our special friends, or we only hold hands with children. When we hold hands, we join together. When you hold your friend's hand you enter into his world and you allow him into yours.

Give your attention to your friend's needs and comfort. Hold hands when it is comfortable for him. Sometimes holding hands takes practice to become comfortable for you!

❋ ⚘ ❋

I recall holding Carl's hand for the first time: I'm driving my car and Carl is riding in the front passenger seat. Carl is becoming agitated and fidgety. His mind is wandering to a focus that is not comfortable. The distance between us seems to grow by the moment. I remember my grandmother reaching out for my hand for comfort while in pain from cancer. Carl is my friend. I want him to have the same love and comfort as Grandma. My stomach is a little queasy and my mind uneasy. I can almost feel sweat beading on my brow. I remember Grandma's love and I reach over and put the palm of my hand on the back of Carl's hand as he taps his thigh. "How are you doing?" I ask as I glance to his eyes with a smile. I gently squeeze his hand. His tight shoulders relax and he turns toward me raising his eyes with a slight look of surprise. His mouth moves slightly into a soft smile.

"OK," Carl responds. Carl's attention begins to wrap around me. I feel somewhat uncomfortable. Carl's thumb begins to slowly rub back and forth against the side of my hand. We are quiet for a couple of minutes. Carl looks at me. "You're a good friend," he says with an affection that stirs my heart.

I look at him and tell him, "*You* are a good friend!"

Carl smiles at me: "Brothers!"

❋ ❦ ❋

The only way you know if holding hands will bring joy to your friend is by taking his hand and looking in his eyes for his response. If he exhibits discomfort, then smile and release his hand. You can also extend your hand toward your friend's hand with your palm upward, toward their eyes. As you do this, look him in the eyes and smile. Then bring your gaze to his hand. This is an invitation for him to place his palm in yours. A third way is to present your hand in the formal gesture of offering to shake his hand. When your friend meets your hand with his, hold it gently. You may also bring your other hand to press against the back of your friend's hand, holding his hand between your two.

Take your time and remember hand holding is a practice of sharing joy. Notice if your friend is receptive. When holding hands is new to your friend, he might not be receptive at first. If this is the case, save holding hands for another day. As your friend progresses on the path of Alzheimer's, a time comes when holding hands is deeply comforting. Holding hands can raise joy in the heart. A state of joy in the heart can be independent of the state of the mind or the brain. Become more and more aware of opportunities for holding hands.

Hand holding is also a way to celebrate a moment of joy. Hold hands whenever it works and feels like a natural expression of friendship. Hold hands when sharing a good laugh, consoling sadness, or walking. Hold hands to dispel uneasiness, to bring your friend's attention to the joy of your friendship, or whenever it is helpful.

Notice how your actions affect your friend's mood. Look for signs in his eyes, the tension of his shoulders, his eyebrows, and the many muscles in the face and neck. Notice the movement of your friend's eyebrows and ears. Notice how your eyes and ears move as you enter new moods.

Always invite your friend's participation with a smile and a feeling of affection. The feelings you hold in your heart will show on the many muscles of your face and neck, and in your posture and gaze. Responding to these emotions does not require cognitive processing, so your friend will be able to understand emotionally. You may even find that as his cognitive abilities decline, your friend's emotional perception becomes more acute.

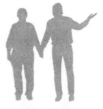

Share His Favorite Food

We have to eat several times a day. Eating can occur and be associated with many memories, emotions, and life events. Food also provides an opportunity to enjoy a variety of colors, textures, tastes, smells, and sounds. These take place in the processes of shopping, preparing, and eating. The key word here is "enjoy!" The opportunity for enjoyment continues beyond swallowing. How you and your friend feel 45 minutes after the meal is of great importance. Does a meal leave your friend with heartburn, tiredness, high energy, or satisfaction? Give every aspect of the eating process the same attention as the taste of the food and regard it with the same importance.

❊ ⚘ ❊

In the small assisted living home where Carl lives, the excitement around food begins when the staff returns from a shopping trip. Residents gather in the living room to watch staff members shuttle past them, moving from the front door to the kitchen in the back of the house. The bustle around the carrying of bags and boxes gets the residents wondering, "What's it going to be this week?"

The staff is cheery. They connect with the residents each time they pass, widening their eyes in excitement. It is apparent this is an important step in creating another week of joy. The mood of the staff creates a level of wonder and excitement.

Each day, excitement begins building before breakfast as the smells of cooking fill the house. The staff is playful, adding various berries to add a splash of color and to make a beautiful presentation that draws raised eyebrows and smiles from everyone. The conversation is much of a replay of words. Every day, Helen comments, "Oh, it looks so pretty!" and Carl laughs in response. More importantly, it is a replay of enjoyment and happiness.

The lunch and dinner preparations are heralded in with the rhythm of chopping and subtle scents of fresh fruits and vegetables wafting in. As residents begin to congregate to see what the next tasty meal will be, snacks are served. Those residents who are able and interested join in the chopping and mixing, taking pride in their contribution. Asking, "What's your favorite?" sparks a lively conversation and makes space for laughter, jesting, reminiscing, and gratitude. The joy of a light and nourishing meal continues with group cleanup, energetic conversation, and enjoyment of time in the yard where trees, flowers, birds, and squirrels engage the senses. Finally, a well-balanced and nourishing meal results in bowels that move easily and regularly, one of the least lauded but most important joys in life.

❊ ⚘ ❊

Enjoy a meal with your friend, either at his home, yours, or at a restaurant he enjoys. Recognize the opportunity for fun in every aspect of the event, from choosing fun clothes to wear, picking a fun route to drive, mulling over the choices on the menu, and talking about his most and least favorite choices.

Go with the flow if your friend's Alzheimer's expresses itself outside the scope of "proper manners". If your friend has difficulty cutting his food, offer to help and smile to express you are happy to be spending this time with him and sharing in the meal. If your friend seems embarrassed, just smile and comment something like, "Sometimes it would be nice if they cut the food in the kitchen!" If he thanks you, just respond, "You're welcome. This is what friends do. We help each other out."

Assisting your friend with eating is a very basic human way to share your love for your friend and make his meal more enjoyable because *you* are with him. In later stages of Alzheimer's, your friend might have trouble using utensils. You can learn to feed your friend when he no longer can feed himself. Many states offer "patient feeding" training programs that are available to volunteers in hospitals, nursing homes and hospices. Contact your state's health department to find out what programs they offer. Sometimes the states don't offer the programs, but regulate their content, delivery, and record keeping, and would therefore be a good source for finding out about programs. You can also contact hospitals, nursing homes, and hospices to find out how they train their volunteers and to learn how you can get the training that is best for you. This training is important because the ability to swallow diminishes in later stages of Alzheimer's and you should know how to respond to your friend's needs so every meal he has with you is safe and enjoyable.

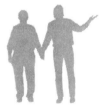

Have a Great Life for Yourself

So, you want your friend to have a great life? Sure! What is the alternative? A not-so-great life. Bummer.... I suggest you choose the great life.

As you spend more time with your friend, you notice the ways her Alzheimer's related symptoms are manifesting. Sometimes she repeats something she just said two minutes previously. This is OK. Just respond anew either the same or differently than the previous time. Have fun with her. Sometimes small accidents or unexpected incidents can cause moments of confusion for her. You can notice at these times how your friend looks to you for the proper way to respond.

For example: Your friend knocks over a glass of water or has an unexpected bladder or bowel release. Before responding with sadness, embarrassment, or laughter, your friend is confused and looks to you for the cue on how to properly respond. In this moment, you determine how this event occurs for your friend. If you respond with shock and dismay, your friend mirrors your feelings as sadness and embarrassment. So, you choose to smile and say, "Hey! This is a good time to get things cleaned up!" Then you help your friend get cleaned up or, if it is convenient, you have a professional caregiver assist.

＊ ⚶ ＊

I'm sitting with Carl and my wife calls me. "Where are you? When are you coming home?" I'm a bit annoyed. And I'm feeling pulled in two directions. This is the first evening in several days that I'm spending with Carl. I want to stay a bit longer. Yet, my wife wants to spend some time with me this evening. I tell her I'm heading home in thirty minutes.

I sit down with Carl and I notice his mood is shifted. He's not as light as two minutes prior. He raises his eyebrows at me. This is his way of saying, "What's up?" He's picking up on my frustration at not being able to be in two places at once. He's suffering with me!

"This is Meredith. She wants me to come home and spend time with her."

Carl laughs and smiles, "Good!"

"I suppose the alternative is that she doesn't want me home. This is actually pretty good!" I laugh with Carl.

I realize: in order to give Carl a great life, I have to have a great life myself. "Carl, I'm going home to see my wife. I'll see you later this week."

"Ha, ha! Good!" Carl chuckles.

When you find it is difficult to "have a great life," look to your family and friends first for support. If you don't get it there, try the resources in the back of this book. Finding a life coach is another way to get the support you want in having a great life. I am available for coaching individuals and organizations. Contact:
David Lazaroff
http://www.joyisavailable.com/coaching
877-926-9300

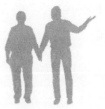

Give a Gift from Nature

Slow your day down and take a look around at the natural world that is always there, ready for your attention to enjoy it. Each season brings variety and gifts. Each day brings growth and shift. Each moment moves without waiting, expressing and sustaining the cycle of life. Intricate details, changing colors, and graceful movements compose the world we live in. The beauty of nature is beyond that which people can manufacture. Such beauty can be soothing, uplifting, and healing.

Select something from nature and bring it to your friend, taking into account any allergies your friend might have. Begin with something for which she has an affinity. Present a flower with a smile and enthusiasm. Marvel with her at the petals, the stem, the stamen, the colors, and the smell. Brush the flower against your face and enjoy the softness. Brush it against your friend's skin and ask her, "Do you like it?" Tell your friend what you like about the flower, steering her attention to the different aspects of its beauty. Have her hold the flower.

Be silent and observe her interacting with the flower and observe her interest. Enjoy your friend's ability to enjoy. See what emotions come up for her. Be content with however your friend interacts with the flower. If she begins to pull it apart, removing petals, let her do so. Let her enjoy the flower in any way she wants to and encourage her interaction.

Consider other natural gifts to present to your friend: a pine cone, a stone, an insect, grass.

❋ 🌿 ❋

Helen's dementia is progressing and she will often ask the same question over and over again. "Where are you coming from? Will you be staying the night?" Helen's heart is welcoming and she is forever the gracious hostess. On Helen's bedroom wall there is a display of colored leaves collected from the ground in autumn. Helen's life is continuously at play with the sights outside her window and the perpetual dance of life in the world around her.

It is mid-October and the leaves are turning and falling from the trees in Denver. As I arrive at the home where Helen is cared for, I stoop to pick up four colorful leaves. I walk into the house.

Helen is sitting in her wheelchair alone at the head of the dining room table. She is thin, small, wrinkled, and beautiful. She wears her favorite sweater. Her hair is neatly pulled back and held in place by a large, colorful butterfly barrette. Her caregivers enjoy her laughter every morning as they bathe and dress her. She appears at rest, her expression is nearly blank. She is very still. Her face is showing boredom. One caregiver is preparing lunch in the kitchen and another is upstairs helping another resident in the bathroom.

"Hello, Helen!" I greet her with a smile revealing my joy at seeing her.

Helen looks up and sees my smile. She raises her eyebrows as the corners of her mouth move toward her ears revealing a white smile. "Well, hello!" she exclaims as she softly slaps her hand on the table to punctuate the moment.

"It's so good to see you." I take the seat next to her and put my right hand on the table next to hers.

"It's good to see you too!" Helen puts her hand on mine and squeezes it. She doesn't remember exactly who I am, but she knows I am a friend. "Are you coming from far away?" Helen asks.

"Not far, just from my job at the Federal Center. The trees are starting to turn with their fall colors. Look what I have for you." I hold my left palm open to Helen. The leaves rest in my palm.

Helen's eyes widen and her mouth drops open in amazement. "Oh my, they're beautiful!" She takes one of the leaves and holds it with both of her hands. "They have so many little veins and features on the edges. And the color reminds me of the color of the forests in the fall in New England."

Helen and I enjoy those leaves for nearly an hour.

Go for a Walk

Whether it is the neighborhood, a park, a school playground, or in a shopping mall, walk in a place your friend enjoys. Go where he likes the things to look at, people to watch, or other enjoyable sights, sounds, and smells.

As his Alzheimer's progresses, going for walks will take more preparation and more time. It's worth the effort! Preparing for the walk is part of what you have to share with him. As you pay attention to the details of getting him ready, he has the experience of your love, concern, and friendship.

Make sure you are prepared for the length of walk you will take, the travel time, and you have everything you need to make it a fun and comfortable trip. A walk around the block does not require as much preparation as a walk in the mall which requires transportation and possible bathroom breaks. It is your business to ask your friend's caregivers what his needs are. Does your friend need assistance in the restroom? Is your friend incontinent of bladder and/or bowel? Do you have the supplies to attend to his needs? Are you comfortable attending to his needs?

Before setting out on an outing of more than a few minutes when your friend is incontinent and requires toileting assistance, practice helping him use the toilet in the home where he is cared for. Get instructions and tips from his caregivers. Be familiar with how to help remove disposable undergarments, clean your friend's bottom and genitals, help him into clean disposable undergarments, and properly dispose of soiled materials. Both you and your friend should be comfortable with this routine before you have to perform it in a handicap accessible stall in the mall or a family restroom at the concert hall. If you're not comfortable with this, bring a caregiver with you on the outing.

❋ 🌱 ❋

Carl needs a new belt, so this is a good time to take him for a walk in the mall. I call his caregivers at the assisted living home and let them know to get him ready.

I walk into the home and Carl is sitting on the couch in anticipation of our outing. "Hey, Carl!" I exclaim.

"Hey, hey!" Carl responds.

Tina, the caregiver walks in from the kitchen. "Is Carl all ready to go?" I ask.

"Yes," Tina answers. "We are done in the bathroom with a bowel movement, so Carl is ready for a few hours."

In my car I have our little travel kit. It is a small

black toiletry bag containing two adult disposable diapers, two pairs of disposable latex gloves, baby wipes, two small plastic bags for containing soiled diapers, wipes, and gloves. We carry this travel kit when we go to any public place. It is small and inconspicuous. I look for the locations of public bathrooms and check for family restrooms that are larger and more comfortable for helping Carl.

We enjoy the ride to the mall, laughing at whatever Carl finds amusing on the road. At the mall we laugh at the belts Carl doesn't like and the ones that are too big and too small. We find one he likes and we buy it.

As we walk in the mall, Carl laughs at a child running back and forth to her parents who sit on a bench. The child shrieks with joy and Carl chuckles and exaggerates a face of pain at the high pitch squeal. "Little stinker," Carl comments.

We sit for lunch and have a couple of slices of pizza and Carl has a cup of his favorite soda. When Carl gets tired of walking, we sit for a few minutes while he recovers his energy.

After about an hour and a half at the mall I ask Carl, "Are you ready to go home."

"Yes."

"Did you have a good time?"

"Yes." Carl's smile is warm, content, and joyful.

Share in His Favorite Music

If you know what kind of music your friend likes, you have an access to sharing his joy of music. If you don't know what kind of music your friend likes, ask him, his family, or his other friends.

There are lots of ways to enjoy music with your friend. One way is to simply sit and listen to the stereo. You can tap your toes, dance with your friend, sing along, mimic the musicians, be dramatic, or just smile and bop your head with the beat.

Join your friend in his world. Notice the feelings the music evokes in him. Play off his joys and just let him go where the music takes him emotionally.

Videos of great musical performances are another way to enjoy time with your friend. If it works to go to concerts, consider it to be a joyful experience of living fully.

❀ ⚜ ❀

I'm at work and the phone rings. It's Carl's number calling.

"Hey, David!"

"Hey, Carl. What's going on?"

"Kris Kristofferson!"

"Kris Kristofferson?" I'm a bit confused.

"Yeah!"

I still don't get it. "OK, Carl. I'll come over after work. Then you can show me."

"OK." Carl hangs up the phone.

After work I knock on Carl's apartment door. He opens the door, motioning me in with excitement. "Here, here, look!"

He hands me the newspaper opened up to a full page ad. Kris Kristofferson is playing in two weeks at the Paramount Theater.

"You like him?" I ask.

"Yeah!" Carl exclaims with certainty.

"Do you want to go?"

"Yeah!" There is not a doubt in his voice.

My mind races with considerations. The tickets are pretty reasonable. However, if Carl likes concerts this could become an expensive habit. We want his money to last in case he lives a long time. Then again, there are no guarantees. He could keel over tomorrow. Every moment of life is truly precious.

A life of joy is about what is available that you like. Carl no longer has a career, no longer can give talks at the meditation center, cannot balance a checkbook or count money, and cannot write letters to friends. Music is available. Carl still enjoys music and recognizes the great artists who compose his music collection and the soundtrack of his life. Getting in and out of theaters is not a problem and bathrooms are accessible.

"OK, Carl! I'll get us tickets."

Over the next two years, until advancing Alzheimer's makes it too difficult for Carl to handle stairs and stay oriented while walking through crowds, we enjoy some of Carl's favorite musical artists who come to town, such as Joan Baez, B.B. King, Eric Clapton, Rod Stewart, Lindsey Buckingham, Bob Dylan, Paul Simon, and Chris Smither.

I let Carl know I appreciate his sharing his love of music with me. I tell him, "If not for your love of music, I would never have the experience of these concerts and the opportunity to appreciate music at this level. Thank you!"

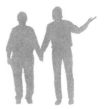

Gaze In Her Eyes with Affection

Sometimes talking with your friend is wonderful. Sometimes the best way to share joy with your friend is in silence. Silence offers us many benefits. If you are not accustomed to silence, take a moment to reacquaint yourself with silence.

Silence is free. Silence presumes nothing. Silence listens. Silence gives space for people to say what they need to say and to hear what needs to be heard. Step into silence and try this exercise with your friend.

When speaking with your friend, complete your speaking and look at your friend's face. Be present with the impact of your friend's life on your life. Recall how she impacts the world of today in her actions and presence from the time of her birth. Connect with why you are with her now. Silently appreciate the kindness she shows in her life, the effort she puts to her work and family, and how her contributions show up in the community. For the moment, look only for that which is beneficial, discarding all else. Fill your heart, your mind, and your emotions with feelings of appreciation for her. Look into her eyes and appreciate what she has seen in life and how she gives you the gift of love and friendship.

When you are joyful about your life and you tell your friend about it, pause for a moment and gaze silently into her eyes, letting your eyes communicate your joy. Listen to her speak her emotions through her eyes. Enter her world and share it as her friend.

❊ ❦ ❊

I walk into the room and Carl is sitting on the couch with his head hanging low. He's not nodding off to sleep. He looks sad. "Hey, Buddy! How ya doin' ?!" My usual cheerful approach is not lifting him out of his doldrums.

I sit next to Carl on the couch. I put my hand on his. He pulls away. He is stuck somewhere in his world. I don't know what is going on in there. I take a deep calm breath and look at the side of his face. The corners of his mouth are drooping. His cheeks are drooping. His eyes gaze downward. His forehead is blank and emotionless. I sense his loneliness.

I recall who Carl is for me. He is an acquaintance turned friend. He is a brother on my spiritual path. He is the receiver of my love, friendship, and joy. He lets me into his heart. As we travel through life together his laugh reminds me the world is a beautiful place when I am looking for beauty. His response to my joy reminds me that how I look at the world impacts how others see it. I am grateful for his gratitude.

A minute passes, and another, in silence.

Carl is not only becoming aware of my presence, but he is becoming curious.

Carl turns his head to see what I am doing, just sitting still next to him. His eyes meet mine. We connect. I smile. Carl smiles.

I raise one eyebrow, "Brothers."

"Yeah," Carl responds. "Brothers!" Carl laughs.

If you want support in being comfortable in the simple intimacies of affection, check out the resources in the back of this book, in particular The Landmark Forum
http://www.landmarkforum.com

Appreciate Him and Tell Him

You're helping out your friend who has Alzheimer's. You help him out a lot. You spend hours visiting, taking him places, making sure he sees the things that make him laugh, and seeing to it that he gets to the weekly service club meeting or place of worship that is important to him for the past 30 years. You are a source of joy and fun in his life. It sure feels good to see your friend smile and benefit from your efforts. It feels good to experience his gratitude and love and to see his life is better for your participation.

Thank him for giving you the opportunity to share your time, love, and life in a way that brings such joy.

There is no opportunity for you to be a giver of love and joy if there is no one willing to take on the job of being a receiver of it. So, thank your friend for letting you into his heart. Thank him for sharing his world with you. Thank him for being a reminder you make a difference that matters.

When you share your appreciation for the relationship you share with your friend, you remind him he adds value to your life. You confirm for him his presence is powerful and his life is valuable. You let him know his contributions are effective and meaningful. Together, you both have a relationship worth celebrating.

❊ 🌿 ❊

After having dinner, watching a movie, playing my guitar and singing, it's time for Carl to go to bed and for me to go home. I put my hand on Carl's knee.

"Carl, it's time for me to go home. I'm having a lot of fun tonight," I say. Carl smiles and raises an eyebrow. "I want you to know how grateful I am to have you in my life. You really make a difference for me." Carl shakes his head in agreement and puts his hand on mine and gives it a squeeze. "Because of you, I have so much more music in my life. Because of you I have the experiences of seeing Bob Dylan, Paul Simon, Eric Clapton, and so many other great artists performing live."

"Yeah, yeah!" Carl bobs his head in agreement.

"You're my friend and I love you."

"Ha, ha, ha!," Carl chuckles.

Tell Her a Secret

We all have secrets. We make them significant and harbor stories in our mind about what other people might think of us if they know our secrets. Keeping something secret keeps others at a distance we think is safe. Sometimes it is wise to keep a secret. Truly, if the wrong person knows, they might wield it recklessly and cause damage that is completely unwarranted.

However, some of the things we keep secret are from times long past and can only cause little or no embarrassment if known by others. In fact, you can look back and laugh in private over them. Surely you can think of a few mistakes in your youth that teach you something, and you just don't want to bring up because it provides no value in the present context of your life. These are the harmless little secrets you can laugh about with your friend who has Alzheimer's. In fact, depending on her ability to remember what you tell her, you may have many opportunities to share the **same secret** with her anew.

If you are visiting your friend and you run out of things to say and you want to engage her, it just might be a good time to tell a secret. Be sure you have enough privacy so no one you don't want to share the secret with can hear it. Also, choose your secret well and consider your friend's ability to repeat the secret and the likelihood she will blurt it out inappropriately.

Open your heart and let her in. Tell a secret that makes you feel a little vulnerable. You can start with, "Hey, do you want to know a secret about me?" If it perks her attention, continue. If you get no response, go ahead and tell her anyway. It is quite possible your friend is taking in much more detail than she shows. I have countless experiences of talking in a room thinking Carl is totally tuned out to everything. Suddenly, Carl breaks out in laughter at what I say. Always treat your friend as if she is listening to you. You never know.

※ ❦ ※

I'm sitting with Carl and he is finished with lunch, I'm out of the songs I usually sing to him, and nothing else is coming up.

"Hey, Carl, can I tell you a secret about me?"

Carl turns his head toward me with a bit of a smirk and one eyebrow cocked. He's game.

"You know, I have a past that includes irresponsible actions I would never do today."

"No shit?" Carl's smirk deepens. It is a typical expression of Alzheimer's patients who become more candid, uninhibited, and a bit crass. He still has his sense of sarcasm. I'm feeling a bit vulnerable and silly at the same time.

"Imagine a kid who has an afternoon newspaper route. He gets home from school late and it is raining. He's tired and just doesn't want to get on his bike and pedal around the neighborhood and deliver those papers." Carl is listening intently with all his attention. "Well that kid is me at eleven years old! So, I push the stack of newspapers from the corner into the storm sewer and blame it on the bullies in the neighborhood!"

Carl is stunned.

"I'm still embarrassed about it more than 30 years later," I continue. "So, Carl, it feels good to get that off my chest." I smile broadly with genuine trust in Carl, "You won't tell anyone my secret, will you?"

"Ha, ha! No, not me!" Carl chuckles.

"I'm glad I'm not that irresponsible kid anymore." Carl is glad too.

BEAUTIFUL MORTALITY!

A Letter to Those Facing the Completion of Life

My Dear Friend,

Great sadness and disappointment are born of hope and attachment to a future that never was and never will be. Waiting for joy in the future or looking for joy in the past denies us of the only source of joy: the present. We only experience love in the present. We only experience laughter in the present. Even our memories are only experienced in the present.

In a blink of time we are born, live our lives, and are gone. There is always one part of the body that malfunctions first. With Alzheimer's it is the brain. Cancer can manifest in any part of the body. From birth, some people live only minutes, others hours, others years, and some live for decades. Very few live more than a century.

Who are we to complain we are mortal? It is our mortality that gives us appreciation and beauty. It is in our mortality that we experience our senses, love, friendship, and companionship. As your disease progresses, your body and your emotions will still respond to touch, music, and warmth. As your brain fails you, celebrate the rest of your being. Surround yourself with love, laughter, and colors. Give the gift of a cheerful countenance to those you love and your love will live on in them after your body is gone. From the dawn of human kind, this is how people live. The names of our ancestors are gone, their worldly deeds are gone, but we still can experience their joy in the language and culture left for us.

Find joy in this world, my friend. Find joy in trees, in animals, in the wind, and in the sea. Find joy in the eyes of your family, in their breath, and in their heartbeats. Search for joy in no moment other than the present. Long for no past or future. The promise of life is here and now and it is beautiful! In a hundred years we remain in the love we live today.

With all my love,
David

The Difference Between
Alzheimer's and Dementia

People at my talks often ask me, "What is the difference between Alzheimer's and dementia?"

According to the Merriam-Webster Medical Dictionary, "disease" is "an impairment of the normal state of the living animal or plant body or one of its parts that interrupts or modifies the performance of the vital functions, is typically manifested by distinguishing signs and symptoms, and is a response to environmental factors (as malnutrition, industrial hazards, or climate), to specific infective agents (as worms, bacteria, or viruses), to inherent defects of the organism (as genetic anomalies), or to combinations of these factors."

A disease is physical: "an impairment of the ... body or one of its parts." If you look at the brain of a person with Alzheimer's disease after their death, you find plaques on the brain that impair nominal functioning.

Dementia is a symptom of disease. When the "vital functions" of the brain are modified in such a manner as to cause wandering, hallucinations, or particular other behaviors or cognitive failures called dementia, these are symptoms.

So, a particular disease has a particular physical

pathology. "Dementia" has no particular pathology. According to the definition of "disease", dementia actually falls into the symptom or expression of the disease; the interrupted or modified "performance of the vital functions ... manifested by distinguishing signs and symptoms...."

In other words, dementia is not a disease, but the signs and symptoms of disease. You will not find dementia in an autopsy. This is why we speak of "Alzheimer's related dementia" or "dementia related to multiple strokes." The disease is Alzheimer's in one case and strokes in the other. The symptom is dementia.

I am available for speaking engagements
domestically and internationally. Contact:
David Lazaroff
http://www.joyisavailable.com/speaking
877-926-9300

Outcomes of Alzheimer's Treatment: What Can We Strive For?

There is very little we can do to treat Alzheimer's Disease. There are many ways we can treat people with Alzheimer's. As you read this, be clear I'm not just talking about Alzheimer's. Alzheimer's is just one path of human health. There are others people travel on without desiring it or planning for it. What is it for you or your loved one? Is it cancer, Parkinson's, Down's Syndrome? Fill in the blank with your disease of choice: We are dealing with

_____.

Whether or not there is a cure for the physical manifestation of the disease, there is treatment for the person.

We have no path to eradicate Alzheimer's from the body. We do have the means to bring joy, love, and comfort to the person with Alzheimer's and their family and friends.

Don't fight it. Don't resist it. Let go of your dreams for a future that will never happen. Reconnect with the purpose of your life. Create a new dream consistent with the physical reality of the disease you are dealing with. Live a life of love and joy.

Let's take this one step at a time.

1. **Work with it.** The usual desired outcome of the treatment of disease is the alleviation of symptoms and the return of function to levels prior to the onset of the condition. With the therapies available for Alzheimer's today, I'm sorry, this is not happening. So, we have to adjust our expectations and create a new vision for the outcomes. We can't turn back the clock to regain the cognitive function prior to the onset of Alzheimer's. We can't stop the progression of the brain deterioration. Perhaps someday, but we can't arrest this disease today. Rivers always flow from the mountains to the sea. Carrying seawater up the mountain will only make you tired; it will not reverse the flow of the river. Today, we have no way to reverse the cognitive decline of Alzheimer's, so let's collect our energy and go with the flow.

2. **Let go of your dreams for a future that will never happen.** You never planned on a life with Alzheimer's Disease, so don't be surprised if your dreams for your future are inconsistent with the presence of Alzheimer's. This attachment to a future that is now inconsistent with the reality of Alzheimer's is the great source of disappointment and sadness that accompanies Alzheimer's. If you have Alzheimer's, you're not going to manage a large investment fund or be the project manager for the construction of a new skyscraper. If your spouse

has Alzheimer's, your conversations are going to be different than they were in your spouse's cognitive years.

3. **Reconnect with the purpose of your life.** Love, joy, beauty, companionship, contribution, and community are always available. Sooner or later we all return to earth, ashes, and dust. When our bodies are spent, we become the raw materials for new life. The purpose of life has not changed since the dawn of time. If your happiness is conditional upon the presence of something that did not exist two thousand years ago, then consider you are disconnected from what is really lasting and nurturing.

4. **Create a new dream consistent with the physical reality of the disease.** Who will share the caring duties? Who will share the love? What do you like? With whom can you do it ? What else will you find to do when the disease process withdraws an activity from your access? This is where those with cognitive abilities must imagine and act for those with Alzheimer's.

5. **Live a life of love and joy.** I prefer love and joy to the available alternatives. You might not choose your physical diseases, but you can choose how you experience your life. You choose what is important in life and to what you give your attention. You can give your

attention to losses and that which you do not have and will never have, or you can give your attention to what is available that you like and in which you find fulfillment. The focus of your attention *IS* your experience of life. I suggest you bring your attention to the love and joy in life. If you don't see it, keep looking. It is there as long as the sun shines and the wind blows. If you don't experience the love and joy in life, then your attention is on other, non-joyful, matters. Finding the joy and establishing yourself in it requires constant effort of the most rewarding kind. Keep at it!

OK, your life is not as easy as reading a book. I suggest you gather with friends, family, and your community. Having a joyful life requires working on finding joy and then working on cultivating joy. It's a big job that is most effectively done with others. Can you think of a better purpose of your life or better outcome than love and joy?

I am available to help individuals, groups, and organizations supporting persons with Alzheimer's, cancer, and other diseases. If you want help in keeping life joyful through all circumstances, call me: Contact:
David Lazaroff
http://www.joyisavailable.com/consulting
877-926-9300

Frail and Laughing

Carl's time in his body is nearing completion. His weight continues to drop from about 230 lbs. a year ago to about 170 lbs. today. His body is bony. He is stooped over when sitting and when standing or shuffling around the room. His words fade between his brain and his tongue. He has two or three gasping attacks in an hour. He has trouble swallowing his food.

I wish him, "Happy New Year!", and Carl laughs. His head hangs low and he appears to not be listening. "Hey, Carl," I call to him cheerfully. He raises his head toward me. His eye is gleaming. There is a deep sparkle from within. He is with me. I put on a New Year's message video of our spiritual teacher, Gurumayi Chidvilasananda, a recording of New Year's Day 2004, and sit on the couch beside him. Carl recognizes Gurumayi's voice. He smiles and laughs in response to Gurumayi's humor.

It is the spring of 2004. Carl receives a diagnosis that the problems he is experiencing since 1997 are the expressions of early onset Alzheimer's disease. When Carl tells me this we shift from acquaintances to friends and I begin helping him.

It is 2011 and Carl's body is nearing the end of its cycle in human form. When this form is complete, it returns to the air and the earth to be absorbed into countless other forms of life. His love, teachings, kindness, and contributions to thousands lives on in those who feel them and are recipients of his 67 years of human life. Then it remains in all their deeds of kindness and in all the people they touch.

"I love you, Carl. I am grateful for your friendship. I am grateful for all you teach me. All your kindness and lessons live in my heart and always will; even the lessons I don't understand fully today. I am grateful Gurumayi and Baba Muktananda bring us together to be friends. You're a very good friend." Carl looks up at me. Our eyes meet. Our souls touch. We recognize we are each other. Life is eternal.

We are two very happy friends. Life is beautiful.

Conclusion

You have a great life. The truth is this world has everything we can possibly want. All the beauty, love, kindness, compassion, and friendship are here. Are you noticing it? To what are you giving your attention?

Enjoy what life offers you with your every breath. A human body is mortal and everybody breathes for a finite period of time. When a body is diagnosed with cancer, Alzheimer's, Parkinson's, or any other dysfunction, do what you can to strengthen the weaknesses expressed in the disease. And, always keep your attention present to the beauty and joy of life. Keep your attention present to what you like and whom you love. Be present to the contribution others make to you and the contribution you make to others.

While we are not always conscious of how we choose our circumstances or how situations come to be, know you have a choice in where you give your attention and how you experience life. Choose love. Choose compassion. Choose beauty. Choose friendship and companionship. Choose joy!

Share your life with enthusiasm. You are a source of joy for everyone you meet. You are a source of joy to the world! Thank you for sharing your love and your joy. You make the world better for everyone.

I am David Lazaroff. My purpose is to help you fulfill your purpose. I want you and the people in your life to have joy, love, and affinity. I'm here for you. Contact:
David Lazaroff
http://www.joyisavailable.com
877-926-9300

RESOURCES

David's speaking calendar is available on
http://www.joyisavailable.com

You can read more of his writings on his blog:
http://blog.joyisavailable.com

For more information about David Lazaroff's
work in creating neighborhood-based
holistic assisted living homes, visit
http://holisticcommunityliving.org

For training in living a life you love and living it
powerfully, go to The Landmark Forum:
http://landmarkforum.com

Online tools to organize your friend's
family and community to share in their care
and the joy of their life:
http://www.lotsahelpinghands.com

For training in Colorado on forming care
communities to share the care for a friend
or loved one who is ill:
http://lifequalityinstitute.org

Learn More!

Visit www.joyisavailable.com for:

NEW PRODUCTS HELPING PEOPLE LIVE GREAT LIVES WITH DISEASE

Including an audio version of "Live It Up! Share a Great Life With Alzheimer's, Cancer, or Any Diagnosis"

❋ ❦ ❋

David Lazaroff enjoys speaking on living a joyful life to audiences of all sizes.

David is available for group, family, and individual coaching. To arrange for a consultation, call David at 877-926-9300 or send an email to david@joyisavailable.com.

David's speaking schedule is posted on http://www.joyisavailable.com

Visit David's other works at:
http://holistic.com
http://holisticcommunityliving.org
http://tomorrowsflowers.com

CPSIA information can be obtained at www.ICGtesting.com
Printed in the USA
BVOW020345170412

287786BV00001B/2/P